FIBER FACTS

GET THE TRUTH CONCERNING DIETARY FIBER

Rita Elkins

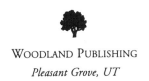

WOODLAND PUBLISHING

Pleasant Grove, UT

Table of Contents

The Great Fiber Famine

Unquestionably, as a society, we are suffering from a deplorable lack of dietary fiber . . . a fiber famine, if you will. And while it is true that we are constantly assaulted with reports and newsflashes warning us that diets low in fiber can literally kill us, for the most part, many of us persist in eating the way we always have. Our diets are chuck full of empty calories, refined foods, loads of sugar and virtually very little in the way of whole foods. When it comes to fiber, too many of us make the mistake of believing that our daily bowl of Wheaties is more than adequate as a source of fiber.

Unfortunately, many of our pantries contain lots of white flour products, cooked and canned vegetables, cookies, chips and all those other brightly packaged foods that make you feel like you've arrived at food utopia. These foods are usually fiberless and have been so artificially altered from their original state, many them are more like "nonfoods."

Typical American eating habits have led to lives plagued with chronic constipation, intestinal gas, bowel disorders, and a whole host of infections. And if we believe that what goes on way down there in our bowel can't be related to our overall health, we're deluding ourselves. The truth is that our ability to expedite waste material from the body is a great predictor of how healthy are. And the fiber content of our food choices determines how that predictor functions. Now, if we want to increase our fiber intake, we must first recognize what fiber is, where its found and how it works. And we must become aware of the profound health impact proper waste elimination has on the human body.

Fiber: A Brief History of Its Demise

Some of our children and some of us, for that matter, would not even recognize certain foods in their whole, natural state. For the most part, whole foods that come form the plant kingdom offer us significant dietary fiber. While food producers and manufacturers have been adding natural and synthetic fibers to foods, they cannot improve on Mother Nature's creations.

Hippocrates, the Father of Medicine, highly recommended eating whole wheat "for its salutary effects upon the bowels." Roman athletes took his admonition to heart and ate whole grains believing that their endurance and strength would be enhanced. Ever since ancient times, whole grains were considered diet staples and were typically consumed by lower class societies who could not afford the fatty, sweet, high protein diets of their king's table.

Unfortunately, progress took a substantial leap backwards when the medical view of fiber was literally reversed in the 18th and 19th centuries. Low-fiber, white wheat flour was hailed as a more available and economical source. Fine sieve roller milling brought white flour home to every table and the fiber famine commenced. What is particularly disturbing is that our fiber-deficient diets are rarely linked to the various symptoms we readily present to our physicians. This was not always so.

Dr. Arbuthnot Lane, who was discovered among Louise Tenney's research on the colon, served as surgeon to the King of England at the turn of the century and spent several years specializing in bowel problems. This medical doctor noticed that after he removed diseased sections of the bowel, his patients experienced remarkable and unexpected cures of completely unrelated diseases, such as arthritis and goiter. These observations caused him to conclude that a causal relationship between a toxic colon and other organs of the body exists. His advice was to care for the bowel first through good, sound nutrition.

Interestingly, certain health advocates in our country protested this view and vigorously tired to promote the merits of bran to the American public. Up until this period of time, fiber had comprised a great part of our diets. Now, fiber-free foods, such as white bread and sugar, were seen as signs of affluence and progress. Dr. J. H. Kellogg, who was none the less still impressed with the value of whole grains, introduced toasted wheat flakes to the nation's breakfast tables in 1895.

It's no coincidence that as our intake of fiber decreased, certain bowel diseases, such as colon cancer and diverticulosis, increased. Ironically, physicians of the 19th and early 20th centuries prescribed the worse possible treatment for these bowel disorders: eating a bland, highly refined diet! Today there are over 85,000 cases of colon cancer diagnosed in our country annually and the number is growing.

In the early 20th century, the science of fiber actually began. The term "fiber" was coined and studies were initiated. Subsequent subjects included the laxative action of bran which was rejected by the American Medical Association; consequently, the publications ceased.

In the sixties, researchers noticed that certain diseases that ravaged our societies were relatively rare in third world communities. Surgeon General T.L. Cleave even went as far as to say that all the diseases of civilization were caused by the "saccharine disease," referring to our blatant over-consumption of sugar and refined carbohydrates.

Fortunately, today, the medical establishment has become more fiber aware; however, unlike the lone voices of the past that tried to extol the virtues of "roughage," they are slow to speak out and even slower to prescribe. We have Cleave, Campbell and Burkitt to thank for their tireless efforts in promoting the consumption of fiber.

Today, we are beginning to rediscover what Dr. Lane already knew: the condition of the colon is intrinsically related to all body systems and can potentially influence numerous chronic diseases, including cancer. Zolton P. Rona, a medical doctor who is acutely aware of this connection has stated: ". . . many degenerative diseases are brought about by toxins generated in the large bowel. Bacterial flora imbalance, putrefaction of undigested foods, parasitic and yeast infections may be at the bottom (excuse the pun) of many diseases." This condition is referred to as autointoxication.

Autointoxication: A Very Real Threat

The frightening array of poisons that an unhealthy colon can harbor is what causes autointoxication. Intestinal toxemia or autointoxication is based on the belief that what you eat determines the kind of bacteria which will inhabit your bowel. For example; if you eat a lot of complex carbohydrates, which are usually fiber rich, and little protein, your intestinal flora will primarily consist of bacteria designed to metabolize carbohydrates. On the other hand, if your diet is high in protein and low in complex carbohydrates, that bacteria will be of the proteolytic type which breaks down and decomposes protein.

This type of bacteria (the bad guys) release harmful gases and toxins which can remain in the colon and find their way back onto the body. Unhealthy intestinal flora can create adverse chemical reactions which can result in the production of powerful toxins. Toxic compounds are created when putrefaction occurs and putrefaction results when the bowel produces harmful bacteria and becomes unable to completely evacuate its contents. The frightening variety of poisons which become trapped in the colon can find their way back into the bloodstream, where the liver has to filter them back out again.

Some of these chemicals are carcinogenic in nature and include compounds such as:

• Bile salts
• Volatile fatty acids
• Heavy metals
• Pigments and preservatives
• Toxins (i.e., phenol, cadaverine, ammonia, creosol, and sepsin)

To make matters worse, we rarely replenish friendly flora by eating good sources of acidophilus (live bacteria). Moreover, we routinely kill our own friendly bacteria by using antibiotics, other drugs, alcohol, etc. In the end, what we create is the perfect habitat for pathogenic bacteria to flourish. Consequently, our colon becomes nothing more than a toxic waste dump. Undigested protein coupled with these poisons has been linked to the development of a whole host of diseases, including autoimmune disorders which have no apparent cause.

One of the best ways to keep yourself colon-healthy is to eat a high fiber diet. Any food material which enters the colon is subject to breakdown by bacterial flora. Dietary fiber reaches the colon intact thereby providing a major source of energy for the intestinal bacteria. In addition, studies have shown that in as little as two weeks, intestinal micro flora can be altered by increasing your intake of dietary fiber. Because dietary fiber affects several vital metabolic processes, eating enough of it is crucial to maintaining good health and preventing disease.

Fiber Decreases Transit Time

Transit time simply refers to how long it takes for what you eat to travel from your mouth, through your stomach and small intestine, to your colon. As mentioned earlier, western nations that eat diets low in fiber have longer transit times than third world countries. It's commonplace for an American to have a transit time of three days to two weeks in cases of severe constipation. Eight to 35 hours is typically seen in cultures where whole grains, fruits and plants are routinely consumed. We must also realize that we can still suffer from constipation even if we consider our selves regular. Cumulative waste which results in incomplete evacuation is a very real disorder. Unfortunately, we have become accustomed to relying on damaging laxatives to prompt what should be a normal physiological function, a problem which can be remedied by simple dietary and supplement additions.

What Exactly is Fiber?

Fiber has been called "roughage" and is technically a food component that remains undigested as it is processed through the gastrointestinal tract. Because it readily absorbs water, it helps to add to the bulk required to form a good bowel movement. Fiber is also described as a complex carbohydrate consisting of a polysaccharide and a lignin substance that gives structure to the cell of a plant. It is the portion of plant food which is not digested. Insoluble fiber has the ability to pass through the intestines intact and virtually unchanged. Unlike fats, carbohydrates and proteins, fiber does not provide the body with nutrients or fuel for energy. It usually has no caloric value. Dietary fiber is found only in plant components, such as vegetables, fruits and whole grains. There are primarily two types of fiber: soluble and insoluble. Some foods contain both types.

Soluble Fiber

Soluble fiber is fiber which will be eventually digested in the large intestine, so its bulking power is limited. Soluble fibers can dissolve in water and have been linked to the following actions:

- Helps prevent blood sugar highs and lows
- Helps lower blood cholesterol
- Lowers the risk of heart disease
- Helps to control high blood pressure
- Encourages friendly bacteria to grow

Insoluble Fiber

Insoluble fiber, which for the most part remains undigested and promotes a faster stool transit time, can:

- Keep the bowel clean and operative and help bind dangerous toxins and hormones for better excretion
- Foster regularity

- Contribute to better digestion
- Prevent constipation
- Help lower the risk of bowel disease

Sources of Soluble Fiber

Soluble fiber is found in pectin, lignin, gums and mucilages and other sources include psyllium, beans, apples, pears, oat bran, etc. This type of fiber usually doesn't seem like fiber. It is digestible and when broken down it creates a kind of gel as it absorbs water in the intestinal tract. Unlike insoluble fiber, this type does not bulk the stool to the extent of insoluble fiber, but it does have a tendency to slow down the rate at which food is digested.

Pectin, gums and mucilage are all soluble fibers and are discussed in a later section. Soluble fiber is found in vegetables, particularly onions, bulbs, leeks and asparagus. Fruits, including dried varieties, are soluble fibers.

Sources of Insoluble Fiber

This type of fiber is primarily composed of cellulose and hemicellulose. Cellulose is a nondigestible form of fiber which is found in the outer portions of vegetable and fruits. It is usually found in their crunchy, woody, stems, stalks, and peels. In addition, the bran or seed covering of whole grains is another type of insoluble fiber. Hemicellulose fibers have the ability to remain unchanged and absorb water as they travel the digestive tract. They increase stool bulk and transit time which both prevent constipation and conditions like hemorrhoids. Stalks, stems, peels and fruit and vegetable skins are all made up of insoluble fiber. Interestingly the insoluble fiber content of fruits is found in its flesh and stringy membranes rather than its peelings.

Total Dietary Fiber

This term refers to the sum of the soluble and insoluble fiber content of a particular food. We need a good variety of foods that contribute to at least 35 grams of dietary fiber to our diet each and every day. Most foods contain both types of fiber. Unfortunately the foods which are the most fiber rich are not usually the ones that are housed in our pantries.

Few families wake up to whole grain cereal, a constant supply of raw fruits and vegetables and the continual consumption of legumes like split peas, beans, lentils or whole grains like millet and barley. Statistics reveal that most of us get 9 grams of fiber per day if we're lucky . . . a statistic that has to change if we plan to live a long and healthy life.

Fiber has the ability to:

- Increase fecal bulk by retaining water
- Decrease stool transit time
- Keep blood sugar levels more stable
- Lower blood serum and liver cholesterol (lipids)
- Help prevent weight gain by slowing the rate of digestion and absorption and help control hunger
- Expedite the removal of potentially dangerous toxins and carcinogens from the bowel by acting as a carrier and by boosting elimination
- Bind with bile salts, which can help decrease the risk of gallbladder disease and certain types of cancer.
- Create the presence of healthier intestinal bacteria

Bran Fibers

The word bran refers to the fibrous covering which surround certain whole grains. Bran is technically referred to as a cereal fiber and is the portion of the grain which was discarded from whole wheat as waste when modern milling processes were established at the turn of the century. Bran has excellent stool bulking capacities and can significantly reduce transit time. To a great degrees, bran was no longer consumed after the introduction of refined flours. It's no coincidence that as bran consumption dwindled, the incidence of certain western diseases escalated. Bran has the ability to hold water better than any other source of fiber. Different cereal brans have their own individual chemical construction and so their ability to retain water can vary.

Oat Bran

Over the last decade, oat bran has enjoyed a high level of publicity, some good, some not so good. When original scientific findings on the benefits of oat bran hit the media, a veritable oat bran frenzy resulted. Technically, oat bran is made by grinding the inner husk of the whole oat grain. Study after study has confirmed that consistently eating oat bran can lower high blood serum cholesterol as much as 20 percent or more. Even already low blood cholesterol can be reduced by 5 percent by consuming daily doses of oat bran. Before we all run out and buy oat bran, it must be understood that it must be eaten consistently and indefinitely to maintain its ability to lower cholesterol. In addition, having a bowl of hot oat cereal and then eating a diet that is high in animal fats is not recommended. Remember that oatmeal, which is the ground version of the whole oat grain contains about one third less fiber than the bran.

NOTE: Be careful not confuse the term "oat fiber" for "oat bran." Oat fiber additions to certain commercial products may originate from oat hulls which is a type of insoluble fiber.

Fiber Intake and American Children

Consciously or not, many of us have been guilty of teaching our kids to turn up their noses at any food that is brown, textured, or speckled. Dr. Oscar Janiger M.D. in his book *A Different Kind of Healing*, referring to a physician who was interested in the healing properties of foods and plants, writes that his interest in the healing properties of foods and plants dated back to the Great Depression, when he was fed whole grains and helped his family grow organic vegetables: "It taught me where foods come from. My parents would take white bread and roll it into a ball and bounce it off the floor saying, this is not food for humans."

A recent study gives us more cause for alarm. Consider the following quote: "Analyses of the U.S. Department of Agriculture's 1977-1978 and 1987-1988 survey data indicate that large percentages (55% to 90%) of children are not meeting minimum fiber intake recommendations established by the American Health Foundation. Mean fiber intakes declined between 1977-1978 and 1987-1988. Fiber from fruits and vegetables declined during this period. . . . Given the importance of fiber in promoting optimum gastrointestinal function in childhood and in treating chronic diseases, such as heart disease, diabetes, and cancer in adulthood, the trends documented in this article are disturbing and suggest that efforts are needed to encourage the consumption of fiber-rich foods among children."

Another study published in *Pediatrics* in 1995 stressed the fact that parents need to become aware of how much fiber their children consume. "Eating fiber-rich foods in childhood promises a whole host of vital health benefits, especially with respect to effective and regular elimination, not to mention its protective role in diseases like diabetes, etc. Until recently, no specific guidelines for dietary fiber intake in childhood are available. A new recommendation for dietary fiber intake has been developed, based on the age of the child, health benefits, and safety concerns. It is now recommended that children older than 2 years of age consume a minimal amount of dietary fiber equivalent to age plus 5 g/d. A safe range of dietary fiber intake for children is suggested to be between age plus 5 and age plus 10 g/d. This range of dietary fiber intake is thought to be safe even if intake of some vitamins and minerals is marginal. It should provide enough fiber for normal bowel activity and may help prevent future chronic disease"

Lack of Fiber Linked to Western Diseases

The Fiber Hypothesis: Burkitt and Trowell, two of the foremost experts on the health implications of dietary fiber, formulated the following hypothesis which is simply that:

- A diet which is rich in foods that contain fiber or plant cell walls (legumes, whole grains, fruits and vegetables) can protect the human body against a wide variety of serious diseases which have specifically attacked western cultures.
- A diet low in fiber or plant cell walls can cause the incidence of these western diseases.

Fiber and Appendicitis

An article in *Gastroenterology*, 1990 states that an increase in appendicitis is prompted primarily by a fall in dietary fiber intake. Appendicitis affects around 200 per 100,000 people every year in the United States. Interestingly, appendectomies are the most common abdominal surgical emergency in the Western world and are comparatively rare in third world countries. While attributing all appendicitis to low fiber diets may be too simplistic, the correlation is clear. It's no coincidence that appendicitis was rare in Western populations until 1870 to 1880 when grains began to be commercially milled and refined and major dietary changes took place. Dr. Burkitt discovered that fiber is the only dietary factor which can significantly speed up the transit of feces through the bowel and lower pressure within the colon. Clinical evidence tells us that when pressure rises in the appendix, it becomes vulnerable to infection by bacteria. Fecoliths or hard lumps of fecal material that obstruct the appendix can certainly occur when the bowel is sluggish, when bowel movements are infrequent, or incomplete or if stool consistency is unformed and dry. A 1940 report explained that when healthy, young Americans added bran to their diets, the appendix, which was invisible before, became visible through barium x-rays. Of further interest is the fact that when diets were forced to revert to more whole grains such as the case in World War II, the frequency of constipation and appendicitis decreased. There is also some evidence that people who get appendicitis may be more prone to develop certain types of cancer, including colon and breast. It may be true that most of us do not find the threat of appendicitis particularly menacing, but its link to fiber is very telling.

Breast Cancer and Its Link To Fiber

Breast cancer is the most common cancer in women. One in every 14 women will develop breast cancer and one in 20 will die from it. Mortality from breast cancer has not experienced a significant change in this century; however, in the 1980s research suggested that deaths can be reduced by a third with regular mammographic examinations. Despite the value of regular screening, the statistics on breast cancer are alarming, to say the least.

Most of us might connect the value of a high fiber diet with cancer of the colon; however, most of us are unaware of its profound role in breast cancer prevention. Several studies have looked into the role of fiber-rich foods in preventing the disease. Twelve case-control studies found a significant decrease in breast cancer risk in women who ate the highest amount of dietary fiber. These studies also found that women who ate the lowest quantity of cereals, beta-carotene, fruits, and vegetables had the greatest risk of developing breast cancer. Keep in mind that the average American woman eats around ten grams of fiber each day.

A 1996 study out of the Oncology Department of St. Thomas Hospital in London concluded that case-control studies conducted in various groups worldwide have reported a correlation between a lower risk of breast cancer with a higher intake of dietary fiber and complex carbohydrates. The study reported, "Although this finding has not been confirmed through American studies, the scope of its observations strongly support the notion that increasing the consumption of fiber or the use of dietary fiber supplements might reduce breast cancer risk in high-incidence populations."

The Estrogen Component and Fiber

Fiber can modify the action of circulating hormones, such as estrogen, which have been linked to the stimulation of certain cancers. In other words, eating fiber helps to rid the body of excess estrogen or undesirable forms of estrogen which can initiate the formation of breast tumors. Eating plenty of vegetable fiber, grain fiber, and fiber from fruits and berries have been associated with low levels of several hormones, including testosterone, estrone, androstenedione and free estradiol. Moreover, many fruits and vegetables contain phytochemicals which can actually inhibit the action of estradiol in women. Cruciferous plants which include broccoli and cabbage contain substances called indoles which can also keep bad estrogen in check. In addition, dietary fiber may also interfere with the development of breast tumors by creating mammary lignins, which are created when plant lignins are chemically changed in the colon by friendly bacteria. Unfortunately, as we've continually stressed, if our colons are compromised, the complete system of defense can break down. Fiber helps decrease transit time, and makes the stool heavier, thereby expediting the removal of cancer-causing substances, including estrogen from the body. Many women are unaware that a significant amount of estrogen is excreted in their bowel movements. Because this waste can sit in the bowel for 24 hours or more, estrogen can be reabsorbed back onto the body. Fiber can help to prevent this phenomenon. Breast cells need estrogen to grow, so if we decrease the amount of circulating estrogen, we decrease our risk of breast cancer.

Fiber works in several ways to prevent estrogen-stimulated cancers:

1. A high-fiber diet reduces circulating estrogen by reducing the recirculation of estrogen through the liver.
2. Most vegetables contain isoflavones and lignins which have the ability to convert into weak estrogens in the bowel that compete with estradiol (bad estrogen) for specific binding sites.
3. A high-fiber diet helps to prevent obesity, which can increase the availability of biologically active metabolites of estrone, a potentially dangerous form of estrogen.
4. Diets rich in fiber and complex carbohydrates have been shown to improve insulin sensitivity while decreasing the amount of circulating estrogen, suggesting a link between these two hormones.

What Kind of Fiber Is Best to Reduce Estrogen Levels?

Several studies have concluded that just increasing your fiber intake may not be as important as what kind of fiber you choose to eat. Scientists have discovered that estrogen levels went down only when sufficient amounts of wheat bran was added to the diet. Because wheat bran is primarily an insoluble fiber this makes good sense. Insoluble fibers can bind much more readily to substances like estrogen. Adding plenty of fresh fruits and vegetables to wheat fiber is also highly recommended.

A Word on All Cancers

There is scientific agreement that three very important dietary goals for the year 2000 should be addressed when it comes to cancer prevention:

1. To increase fruit and vegetable consumption to 5 or more servings every day
2. To increase breads, cereals, and legumes to 6 or more servings daily
3. To decrease fat to no more than 30% of total calories.

Current data suggests that these goals will not be effective based on past behavior. Unfortunately, just emphasizing the important of dietary changes in conjunction with recommending annual medical tests has not been embraced by the public as anticipated. Predictions tell us that without adequate education and implementation strategies for dietary changes in the general population, patterns will continue or worsen. It is thought that by changing our diets we could prevent more than 300,000 new cases of cancer each thereby preventing 160,000 deaths, and saving $25 billion in associated costs.

Cholesterol Levels, Heart Disease, and Fiber

More recently, attention has focused on natural ways to bring down cholesterol levels, and fiber use is at the top of the list. Did you know that fiber supplementation in the form of psyllium can bring down high cholesterol levels? A 1987 article published in the *Journal of Cardiology* states that LDL or bad cholesterol levels can be reduced by as much as 22 percent by using psyllium and bean fiber sources. In addition, new findings state that soluble fiber can reduce the risk for coronary heart disease by more than 30 percent. It can actually cause a decrease in high blood pressure. In a more recent trial examining the effects of dietary soluble fiber supplementation, total serum cholesterol and LDL cholesterol fell on average by (-14.9%) and (-17.9%) respectively, while HDL cholesterol increased (+30.1%). Serum triglycerides decreased (-30.7%) and the cardiovascular risk ratio (LDL/HDL) fell by (-36%). Total cholesterol reduction was seen as low as (-45%) with LDL decreasing as low as (-59%) and HDL increasing as high as (+48%). Clearly, fiber supplementation is a safe, effective, natural way to lower cholesterol and should be used alone or in conjunction with other therapies.

Using it can reduce your risk of heart disease. A 1994 study found that a low-fat, high-fiber diet may not only reduce the incidence of atherosclerosis but may also lower an individual's risk of developing a blood clot.

Here are some important facts to know:

1. Sources of soluble fiber can significantly reduce your risk of heart disease. These include dried beans of all kinds, lentils,

split peas, oat bran, rice bran, barley, psyllium, gums and pectins (wheat fiber, cellulose and lignin are not as good, however they speed transit time which can also remove excess cholesterol and lipids from the body).

2. Soy fiber has also shown promise in preventing arterial disease.
3. Fiber reduces cholesterol levels in a number of fascinating ways:
    a. It delays the emptying our of stomach contents which results in less fat absorption.
    b. It speeds transit time, which affects the breakdown and absorption of fats
    c. It affects enzyme function from the pancreas which results in separating enzymes from fats which changes the way they breakdown.
    d. Fiber alters the flow of lymph which affects the rate in which fats enter into the circulation from the digestive system
    e. Fiber influences the secretion if insulin which has a bearing on how lipids are broken down in the bloodstream and stored.

Colon and Colorectal Cancer

Colon or colorectal cancer refers to malignant tumors or lymphomas of the large intestine or rectum. Because these types of cancer are considered western diseases, the role of diet is extremely important. A high-meat, high-fat and low-fiber diet encourages the production and concentration of carcinogenic substances in the bowel and rectum. A genetic predisposition to the disease also plays a role. In 1987, 60,00 Americans died from cancers of the colon, rectum and anus and around 145,000 new cases were reported. In 1994, 70,000 men and 67,500 women were diagnosed with colon and rectum cancer. The National Cancer Institute predicted that 6 percent of 250 million U.S. citizens would eventually develop colon cancer and six million of them would die from it. There is perhaps, no disease which could benefit more from fiber than colon and colorectal cancer.

Here's an interesting finding. A study discussed in a 1990 issue of *Cancer Research* states that fat has no effect on colon cancer development when dietary fiber content is high. What this implies is that fiber increase may be more important that fat decrease when it comes to preventing colon diseases. A 1992 study published in the *Journal of the National Cancer Institute* found that rates of colorectal cancer in various countries are strongly correlated with per-capita consumption of red meat and animal fat and inversely associated with fiber consumption.

Consider this statement made by Richard Passwater in his book *Cancer Prevention and Nutritional Therapies:*

> *"The vast majority of human colon cancers are due primarily to the chemicals that are by-products of the decomposition of bacteria and excess dietary fat and bile in the colon. A low fiber diet contributes to colon cancer by slowing down the system so that these decomposition products linger in the colon for extended periods. This increases the length of time that these decomposed products are in contact with the colon and increases the amount that is absorbed into colon cells."*

Eating fiber helps to promote the cultivation of good bacteria which means that the number of bad bacteria will decrease is vital to understanding how to maintain our health. The state of hour health is determine to a great degree by the kind of bacteria which inhabit our colon. Eating fatty meats, refined sugar and low fiber generates putrefactive bacteria which produce harmful, carcinogenic compounds.

What is really interesting is that when we balance out our diets with certain foods, even if we eat high fats, we are afforded a certain amount of protection from developing colon as well as other cancers. Cultures like the Finns who eat a high fat diet but combine it with lots of fiber and active culture yogurts have a low incidence of colon cancer. In addition, one clinical study interviewed over 600 people with colorectal cancer compared with 3000 members of a control group and found that colorectal cancer patients consumed less fruit, vegetables and cereals than the controls. The double whammy of a low fiber diet as it relates to colon cancer can be summed up by these two actions.

1. Low fiber eating means producing bad bacteria which generate carcinogenic compounds in the colon
2. Low fiber eating means harboring those compounds for long periods of time before they are expelled from the body

Eating plenty of wheat bran or other types of cellulose can reduce our risk of colon cancer. It's that simple. Emphasize whole grains, like wheat and barley and eat plenty of legumes like dried beans, split peas, lentils. Oat bran, guar gum and raw fruits and vegetables are also excellent.

Constipation

Hippocrates, the father of medicine held that for the maintenance of good health, defecation should occur "twice or thrice" daily. Today, answers range from after every meal to four times per week. Generally speaking, if you have less than four bowel movements per week and if those movements are unformed or difficult to pass, you can consider yourself constipated. Many natural health care advocates define constipation as anything less than one bowel movement per day. More women suffer from constipation than men.

Constipation is really more of a symptom that an actual disease. Technically speaking, constipation refers to a decrease in bowel movements or difficulty in passing the stool. In some cases, diarrhea can be considered a form of constipation. Constipation can lead to diverticular disease and hemorrhoids, not to mention a wide variety of ailments linked long transit times and poorly formed stool. Recently the notion that you can have regular bowel movements and still be constipated has received more attention. This idea is based on the incomplete evacuation of the bowel even when bowel movements are frequent. This implies that waste residue builds up on the colon walls and is not properly excreted with the movement of bowel muscle. In other words, it sticks and can create toxins and other bowel disorders. In the United States alone, annual sales of laxatives and stool softeners amount to $500 million per year.

Adding fiber to your diet, especially wheat bran can help prevent and get rid of chronic constipation. The amount of fiber recommended for anyone who suffers from constipation is 40 grams per day. Remember that all wheat brans are not equally effective. Coarse bran is better. Cereal sources of fiber are better for constipation that fruit and vegetables, however a combination of these foods is ideal. Eating foods like wheat or oat bran must become part of a daily routine in order to treat and prevent constipation. Adding a psyllium supplement can move things along if your diet is lacking. Learn to routinely eat figs, prunes, watermelon, carrots, sesame and sunflower seeds, and berries. Most importantly, eat whole grains and don't forget the bran.

Diabetes and Hypoglycemia

There is compelling data that fiber-depleted diets that are typically high in refined, processed foods have greatly contributed to the development of diabetes in our society.

Approximately two people for every 1000 have type one diabetes by the time they are 20 years old. Type two diabetes affects an estimated 5.5 million Americans. Around 2000 people for every 100,000 are affected. We know that consuming sugar is certainly an important factor in causing this disease, however, the amount of fiber consumed along with that sugar may even just as crucial. If carbohydrates like maize or millet are eaten in their whole form which is high in dietary fiber, blood sugar levels rise much slower.

In 1942, when cereal shortages necessitated the introduction of high fiber flour to replace white flour, diabetes mortality rates began to fall and continued to do so until 1954. By the mid 1970s a number of clinical studies had already concluded that increasing the amount of fiber consumed has a desirable effect on diabetics.

Fiber slows the absorption of food in the small intestine. The rate in which carbohydrates are digested is closely related to how fast they are absorbed which determines the rise of blood sugar. When carbohydrate and plant fibers are eaten together, blood sugar levels are considerably lower that when the same type of carbohydrate is eaten alone.

The fact that so many people suffer from what is referred to as hypoglycemia testifies to the fact that we are bombarding our bodies with simple sugars without the benefits of fiber. Hypoglycemia indicates an overly stimulated pancreas which can eventually lead to its demise resulting in diabetes. The average American consumes over 125 pounds of white sugar every year. Sugar makes up 24 percent of our daily calorie intake, with soda pop supplying the majority of sugar. As a nation we eat an average of 15 quarts of ice cream per person per year. Our diets are loaded with sugar, hidden or added from our first bowl of sugary cold cereal to our daily big gulps, pastries, chips and candy bars.

To compound the problem, we have fragmented foods, fruits, grains, etc., which further hampers our ability to metabolize glucose. Laboratory studies have confirmed the bad news: removing fiber from food or physically disrupting it disturbs glucose level stability and enhances insulin response which results is rebound hypoglycemia. In other words, if you drink large quantities of apple cider instead of eating a whole apple, who can shoot your blood sugar sky high, which creates a surge of insulin which brings it down to a quick low, which makes you desperately crave more sugar so the vicious cycle propagates itself. Guar gum has also proven itself as a blood sugar lowering fiber.

What Fiber Can Do for Diabetes:

- Reduce the amount of insulin needed by keeping blood sugar levels lower
- Lower cholesterol and lipid levels in the blood which can become elevated in the presence of too much insulin.
- Help to promote weight loss which can even cure some cases of adult onset diabetes

Gallstones

Did you know that the highest incidence of gallstones is found in animals with the lowest fiber intake? Gallstones form when cholesterol crystallizes with bile in the gallbladder. Between one and ten stones may collect in this small sac and symptoms may not occur until one of the stones becomes stuck in the bile duct. The alarmingly high incidence of gallstones in the United States is directly related to western dietary habits (where have we heard that before?) A high-fat, high-protein, refined-carbohydrate diet which elevates blood cholesterol levels increases the risk of developing gallstones. The fact that gallbladder removal surgery is one of the most common operations in the United States fives us some idea of how prevalent gallstones are. Over 20 million people suffer from gallstones, with at least 1 million new cases diagnoses each year.

In the 1970s a hypothesis was presented that eating refined, fiber poor foods supercede the liver's ability to make bile acids which resulted in less bile. The less bile, the more the contents of the gallbladder stagnate . . . the more stagnation, the higher the risk of stone formation. The addition of cholesterol-rich foods only compounded the problem elevating lipids in the gallbladder which became bound to the bile acids and formed more stones. Now, to really make matters worse, if waste material stayed in the colon too long, toxic bile acid metabolites were reabsorbed into the body, causing the production of bile to be further impaired.

The story doesn't end there . . . if you eat a fiber-depleted, refined-carbohydrate diet, you have a tendency to become obese which increases cholesterol synthesis. And here's the clincher . . . the incidence of gallstones is related to coronary heart disease, diabetes, obesity, diverticular disease hiatal hernia and cancer. Everyone of these diseases can be linked to low fiber, high fat diets. Simply put, fiber-depleted foods are a risk factor for gallstones.

Scientific studies with animals have confirmed that the highest incidence of gallstones is found in animals who ate low fiber diets. Dietary fiber:

- Reduces bile cholesterol concentrations
- Keeps the bile acid pool active which discourages the formation of stones
- Helps to prevent obesity which is significantly lined with gallbladder disease
- Helps to bind with toxic bile acid metabolites in the colon keeping them from being reabsorbed into the bloodstream

Supplementing the diet with fiber, such as wheat bran, can help to leach out cholesterol form the liver as it crosses the portal blood to the bile.

NOTE: The types of fiber that have been tested for their effect on the gallbladder include wheat bran, lignin fibers and barley fiber.

Hemorrhoids

A hemorrhoid is nothing more than a varicose vein located in the anal region. These distended veins can swell and protrude causing pain and itching. Repeatedly straining to move hard dry feces typically causes hemorrhoids although they can occur as a complication of pregnancy and child birth. It has been estimated that approximately one in two Americans over the age of 50 suffers at some time or another from hemorrhoids. A low-fiber diet causes the stool to become unformed, hard and dry. Straining during a bowel movement causes venous pressure to rise, making veins more vulnerable to injury. When you have to force a bowel movement, delicate mucous membranes can become damaged. These abrasions and swollen veins can bleed, causing all kinds of discomfort.

A lack of fiber, especially cereal fiber can cause the formation of hard feces. Eating high fiber foods or using vegetable based fiber supplements result in a soft, formed stool which can pass easily without straining. Additional studies have confirmed that adding bran to the diet improves stool bulk, decreases transit time, encourages the healing of hemorrhoids and discourages their recurrence. In addition, if you're treating your hemorrhoids with medications or recovering from a hemorrhoidectomy, you'll recover sooner if your boost your fiber intake.

Fiber and Irritable Bowel Syndrome

A few years ago, doctors prescribed bland diets for anyone suffering from colitis or irritable bowel syndrome. The notion that high fiber could help an irritated colon that vacillated from constipation to diarrhea didn't seem plausible. Today, medical doctors have finally realized that high fiber diets and bulk-forming agents can effectively treat these types of colon disorders. Using bran or substituting whole meal bread for white bread resulted in a significant improvement in symptoms of people with irritable bowel syndrome.

Gentle natural laxatives such as Citrucel are routinely prescribed by doctors for colitis. Some doctors have even used psyllium therapy although the citrus based laxatives are considered somewhat more gentle. Clearly, while eating oat bran may not provide an overnight cure for an inflamed colon, it will eventually result in a much healthier one. The question as to why the colon became inflamed in the first place is rarely addressed by the medical establishment.

Anyone who gulps their food, has high stress levels and eats a low fiber diet is putting a great deal of pressure on their colons. Sufficient chewing activates enzymes in the saliva which helps to digest food properly. The highly sweetened cold cereal, soda pop, hamburger and french fry diet can lead to fiber depletion and colon irritation.

Pectin fibers (found in apples and other fruits) are particularly good for an inflamed colon and should be eaten liberally. Bulking up the stool is also great for both the constipation and diarrhea than come with colitis and irritable bowel syndrome.

It's important to gradually switch to high fiber foods so that the colon can adjust. Be careful with popcorn . . . it can promote diarrhea and should not be eaten until the colon heals. Start with $1/2$ cup of oat or wheat bran cereal and go from there. Work yourself up to $1 1/2$ cups every day and add lots of raw fruits and vegetables.

Prostate Cancer

Prostate cancer occurs when a malignant growth forms in the outer zone of the prostate gland. Unfortunately, the symptoms of prostate cancer can be rather vague. Consequently, approximately 90 percent of prostate cancer goes undetected until it has progressed to a much more serious stage which is difficult to treat. Developing prostate cancer has been linked to several factors; however, its dietary connection has recently been strengthened. What men choose to eat has a profound effect on their prostate health status. In addition a history of venereal disease, and chronic prostate infections have also been associated with an increased risk of prostate cancer. Statistics indicate that 103 men in one thousand will develop prostate cancer. In 1993, 132,000 men were diagnosed with prostate cancer and 34,000 of them died from it. The incidence of prostate cancer has escalated by 39 percent since 1973. Fiber helps to prevent this cancer much the same way it works for breast cancer prevention. An article in the *Journal of Steroid Biochemistry* states that "fiber intake protects against prostate cancer."

Obesity and Fiber

When it comes to weight loss, fiber offers us a veritable panacea of desirable effects. A diet that is high in fiber that emphasizes plenty of whole grains, raw fruits and vegetables and is lower in protein and fats can help to meet the criteria listed above. We live in an incredibly prosperous society and rarely deny ourselves the vast array of fattening delectables that surround us on every side. We need to redirect our notions of what is appetizing or appealing foods and reach for unrefined, whole, nutritious foods.

So, how are we doing? Data published by the Nationwide Food Consumption Survey (NFCS) in 48 states with 9027 individual adult men and women evaluating dietary intake over a three day period found that typically Americans consumed more calories from total fat than recommended, and that they continued to consume lower intakes of fiber. Despite media reports and publications on the profound value of fiber, fiber intake did not change. Interestingly while fat consumption did decrease on the whole, the incidence of obesity rose suggesting that the glut of low-fat or no-fat foods available on our grocery store shelves has done little to further our weight goals. To the contrary, eating a lot of low fat, high carbohydrate foods that are low in fiber can actually promote weight gain.

Various 1990 studies found in the *International Journal of Obesity* stated that "dietary fiber has proved beyond all doubt to be of value in the management of the overweight, in helping weight loss and in shrinking hunger feelings. In addition, the greater your fiber intake, the higher your waste of calories will be. Energy output is increased with the bulking action of fiber. Dr. Burkitt, one of the leading experts on dietary fiber believes that the type of obesity common to western cultures is profoundly linked to the fact that our calorie-rich diets are fiber poor. Fiber is the only constituent that we eat that is calorie free. Consequently, if a high fiber diet can actually decrease the energy we absorb, it seems reasonable to assume that a fiber-rich diet will help to keep a person slim.

Specific Actions of Fiber that Promote Weight Loss

Fiber can control weight in various ways such as:

- Increasing saliva production
- Increasing chewing time
- Increasing gastric filling
- Slowing gastric emptying
- Slowing glucose absorption
- Lowering insulin secretion
- Increasing fecal excretion

The Colon's Connection to Weight Loss

The status of our colon is rarely linked to obesity. The fact that weight reduction can be significantly inhibited by chronic constipation must be recognized. Here we go again: cultures that routinely eat high fiber diets have a very low incidence of obesity. Unquestionably, these people do not count calories to maintain their ideal weight.

Fiber reduces the absorption of fat by drawing water into the intestinal system which creates a sensation of fullness with less caloric intake. Studies have found that when high fiber diets are consumed over a period of time, food cravings will diminish.

Dietary fiber can prevent and treat obesity by:

- Slowing down the eating process by increasing the amount of chewing required.
- Increasing the excretion of fat in the feces.
- Improving digestive hormone secretion which facilitates better digestion and reduces food intake.
- Improving glucose tolerance to prevent wild blood sugar swings.
- Creating a feeling of fullness or satiety.

Fiber Supplements and Weight Loss

Using a good fiber supplement is highly recommended as a way to ensure that you're getting adequate amounts of soluble and insoluble dietary fiber. The best kinds of supplements utilize a combination of pectins, gums and brans. In relation to weight loss, psyllium has an impressive track record. Because it is such a good bulking agent, psyllium supplements can significantly boost the process of weight loss.

In Italy, a study on the effects of Plantain (psyllium) in a reducing diet for women who averaged about 60 percent overweight resulted in weight loss greater than that obtained by diet alone. The effects of psyllium on weight loss was dramatic. In summary, it appears that psyllium produces weight loss by limiting caloric intake, due to its appetite-satiating effect, and by reduced intestinal absorption of lipids.

Taking a daily dose of a fiber supplement can expedite weight loss by:

- Increasing your feeling of fullness and discouraging food cravings and abnormal hunger surges.
- Providing intestinal bulk which helps to clear lipids from the body without contributing one single calorie in the process.

Varicose Veins

Varicose veins are vessels which have become swollen due to a weakness in the vein wall or valve, allowing a backflow of blood to occur. As a result, blood pools in superficial veins, causing them to become stretched and puffy. The legs are more susceptible than any other area to varicose vein development. Spider veins, which are usually found in the thighs are a much milder form of varicose vein. Varicose veins can be aggravated by a lack of good circulation which results in the twisting and dilating of veins. Pregnancy, or prolonged standing have been associated with the development of varicose veins. It's important to understand that these component are secondary not primary causal factors. In other words, while certain situations make it easier to generate varicose veins, other, more important reasons determine their existence.

More than 40 million Americans suffer from varicose veins, with women outnumbering men four to one. Varicose veins are one of the most common disorders that surgeons confront and the prevalence of them is rising. Varicose veins are seldom seen in areas of the world where high-fiber diets are the rule. Typical western dietary habits unquestionably contribute to the development of varicose veins.

Dr. Burkitt questioned doctors in over 200 hospitals in nearly 50 countries and found that the incidence of varicose veins was practically zero in Asia and Africa. Again, the more affluent the community, the greater the incidence of the disorder. The main factor that affected the prevalence of varicose veins in these communities was the degree of contact with Western civilizations. Dr. Burkitt concluded that if pregnancy or standing too long caused varicose veins then the malady would be evenly distributed throughout the world. In fact he postulated that there should be less varicose veins in western cultures, where people could sit more throughout the course of a normal workday.

Burkitt discovered that communities with very low incidences of varicose veins were the same ones who consistently had healthy and ample bowel movements. He concluded that when we get constipated, intra abdominal pressure rises which can cause abdominal straining. The one, most important cause of constipation so prevalent in the western world was a lack of cereal fiber in the diet.

How Much Fiber Do We Need?

A good diet should include 25 to 35 grams of fiber or at least 1 ounce of dietary fiber each and very day. Some health practitioners are recommending up to 50 grams of fiber per day. Two thirds of that fiber should be insoluble. Adding wheat bran to your diet is the easiest way to boost your fiber intake. The average American eats from 9 to 13 grams of fiber per day. The ideal barometer of determining if you're getting enough fiber is whether you have a good bowel movement at least every 24 hours. Your transit time is very important. Unless you suffer from certain bowel conditions like Crohn's Disease or ulcerative colitis some experts believe that you can't get too much fiber.

How To Boost Your Fiber Intake

- Add fiber gradually.
- Drink plenty of water.
- Chew your foods thoroughly so that the necessary digestive enzymes to digest the food will be activated in the saliva.
- Take a digestive enzyme supplement with meals.

Many of us mistakenly think we're getting enough fiber through our diet. Let's go over foods from worse to best in fiber content.

Foods which contain no fiber:
Dairy products (milk, cheese, yogurt, sour cream, buttermilk, etc.)

Foods with a relatively low fiber content:
Leafy vegetables (lettuce, cabbage, watercress, etc.), some fruits

Foods that have a moderate fiber content:
Root vegetables (beets, turnips, carrots, potatoes, parsnips, yams)

Foods that are high in fiber:
Legumes (split peas, dried beans, lentils), seeds, nuts and dried fruits (especially figs, dates, and prunes).

Foods that have the highest fiber content:
Whole grains (wheat, oats, millet, rice, corn, barley, and buckwheat)

Can you see why eating a lettuce salad everyday is not a good source of dietary fiber. Salad bars are great; however they do not usually provide enough dietary fiber. Adding garbanzo or kidney beans, corn, whole wheat, broccoli, carrots, and beets can raise the fiber value of your salad. Learn to spot fiber-friendly veggies and add them liberally. Remember that just because a vegetable looks stringy or "fibery" doesn't mean that it is.

Can You Get Too Much Fiber?

While this subject spawns considerable debate, some healthcare experts believe that eating more than 35 grams of fiber per day is not a good idea. They believe it may adversely affect vitamin and mineral absorption. While this is technically true, it is rarely the case because most of us eat nowhere near the amount of fiber we need. Cultures that routinely eat 60 grams of fiber per day are not necessarily vitamin or mineral depleted and can be considered well-nourished.

While it is true that some fibers may absorb calcium, zinc, iron and magnesium and that the presence of fiber in the intestines may inhibit the absorption of certain fat-soluble vitamins, these effects are present only under extreme conditions. In other words, don't let the fear of becoming nutrient deficient stop you from boosting you fiber intake. This particular phenomenon does not pose a significant threat. The marvelous benefits of fiber far outweighs the very remote possibility that you will eat quantities large enough to pose any problem.

Simple and painless ways to increase your fiber intake:

- Take a good fiber supplement every morning with your breakfast or 30 minutes before any meal.
- Grab a handful of oat cereal when you get the urge to snack.
- Add bran, millet, barley, etc., to your meatloaf, casseroles, pancakes, cake and cookie batters, stuffings, and compotes.
- Use crunchy granola cereals or barley nuts as a topping for ice cream, yogurt, baked potatoes, fish, salads, etc. Adding whole wheat that has been soaked to salads is delicious. Always add seed or fresh raw fruit to make yogurt more fiber acceptable, and only buy active culture yogurts.
- Eat fresh, raw fruit and vegetables with their peelings whenever possible.
- Reach for prunes, dates, or figs when you need to appease your sweet tooth instead of cookies, candies or juice.
- Look for fiber-rich foods offered in salad bars and add them liberally (brachial, carrots, red beans, garbanzo beans, sunflower seeds, etc.)
- Get in the habit of sprouting your own legumes. Peas, lentils, mung beans, garbanzo beans, lentils, soybeans, wheat, etc. can all be sprouted and make delicious additions to tossed green salads.
- Buy canned, precooked beans of all kinds and add them to salads, soups, casseroles and stews.
- Keep a good supply of grains on hand that you can add to any recipe to make it more fiber-rich. Good grains are millet, barley, brown rice, whole oats and whole wheat.

Foolhardy Fiber Sources

- Watch out for terms, names or appearances which you may assume are signs of high-fiber foods

- Brown colored breads, rolls, cookies, etc. are not necessarily high in fiber. Caramel coloring is frequently added to food products to make them appear more appealing or natural.
- Terms such as "wheat," "wheatberry," "multigrain," "natural," "fortified," etc., do not mean that the whole grain has been used. Many products with these kinds of names are mostly comprised of white flour. Even the term "whole wheat" doesn't necessarily mean that all of the flour used has been milled from the whole grain.
- Watch out for naughty, high-fat, baked good which are disguised as fiber rich foods. Oat bran doughnuts, cookies or even tortilla chips are commonly high in fat and sugar and notoriously low in oat bran. A *New York Times* survey showed that some "oat bran" muffins contain so little oat bran that they are virtually useless as a source of fiber. For example, a single bran muffin can contain as much fat as 3 lunch size bags of potato chips. Just because it has bran in it, doesn't necessarily make it good for you. The use of coconut oil, hydrogenated vegetable fats, linseed oil, etc., have all been linked to coronary artery disease.
- New varieties of snack crackers that sound fibery are really nothing but doctored up white flour foods. Many whole grain saltines, wheat crackers, etc., fall into this category. Always check for fiber content and ingredient listing.
- Nuts can be a good source of fiber but they usually come salted, processed and are often rancid. Look to buy raw nuts, preferably unshelled such as almonds, pistachios, etc.
- Just because something is crunchy or requires chewing doesn't mean it has a high fiber content. Celery is one of those tough vegetables that is all crunch and low fiber.

Fiber Supplements Can Lifesavers

Because most of us have good intentions but rarely meet our optimal dietary goals, fiber supplementation is recommended. Ideally, we should be eating enough "fibery" foods in the form of raw fruits, vegetables, and whole grains. Realistically, we usually fall short, no matter how dedicated we might be. If we have any type of glucose impairment disorder like diabetes, we may not be able to eat the amount of fruit recommended, or we may never develop a taste for whole grain cereals, or may consistently skip meals. Moreover, if we are allergic to grains like wheat, obtaining enough fiber could be significantly more difficult. For this reason, a good, vegetable-based fiber supplement can be extremely desirable. The advantages of taking a good fiber supplement include:

1. Its an easy way to fortify your diet with fiber two to three times a day if desired.
2. Vegetable fibers that have been ground to powders can make the fiber source more digestible
3. Fiber formulas can contain sources of fiber as well as other nutrients or herbs that we would normally not consume like guar gum, pectin, psyllium, etc.
4. Fiber supplements sometimes contain a variety of fiber sources which are much more preferable than just one fiber food. Different types of fiber initiate different physiological responses in the human body.
5. Fiber supplements can be taken anywhere (trips, camping, etc.).
6. Taking a fiber supplement on a daily basis helps to lower cholesterol levels, speed transit time and prevent constipation, and contributes to weight management.

Fiber supplements are usually available in powder form and are designed to mix with a liquid. They are typically blended into juices, hot cereals, casseroles, dressings, and gravies. if you find them difficult to take in drink form, think of creative ways to sneak them into moist food like batters (pancake, waffle, cookie, cake, etc.), soups or stews.

NOTE: Experience has proven that if you add fiber supplements to your diet, they work better if you rotate them. Popular and effective supplements include gum acacia, pectin, guar gum, oat fiber, psyllium seed, apple pectin, agar and flaxseed. For optimal results, make sure you get adequate amounts of fiber preparations.

Take your fiber supplement 30 minutes before you eat to help curb your appetite and create satiety and drink plenty of water.

Remember that you need to take fiber supplement for at least three months to begin to consistently see physiological benefits. Begin to add fiber slowly to your diet and try not to overdose on just one type of fiber. Fiber formulas that include a variety of fiber or a mix of vitamins, herbs or minerals are especially good.

Summary

Today, we know the facts. We can't claim ignorance to justify our food choices. Fiber can significantly deter potentially fatal disease, contribute to weight control and profoundly improve our health and well being. Fiber supplementation is one of the easiest and simplest additions we can make to our diet which pays us back with incredibly high health dividends.

References

Andersson, H., et al., *Human Nutrition: Applied Nutrition,* Apr. 1985, 39A: 101.

Bal, D.G., and S.B. Foerster, *Cancer,* Aug 1, 1993, 72(3 Suppl):1005-10.

Banji V; Betts N., "Fat, cholesterol, fiber and sodium intakes of US population: evaluation of diets reported in 1987-88 Nationwide Food Consumption Survey. *European Journal of Clinical Nutrition,* Dec. 1995, 49(12):915-20.

Birch, G.G., and K. J. Parker, *Dietary Fiber,* (London: Applied Science Publishers, 1983),

Dreher, Mark L., *Handbook of Dietary Fiber,* (New York: Marcel Dekker, Inc., 1987).

Hoover-Plow, J., et al., "The glycemic response to meals with six different fruits in insulin-dependent diabetes using a home blood-glucose monitoring system," *American Journal of Clinical Nutrition,* Jan. 1987, 45(1): 92-7.

Jenkins, D.A., et al., "Treatment of Diabetes with guar gum: Reduction of urinary glucose loss in diabetics," *Lancet,* 1977, 2:779.

Keitch. G.J., et al., "Dietary fiber and giardiasis: dietary fiber reduces rate of intestinal infection by Giardia lamblia in the gerbil," *American Journal of Tropical Medicine and Hygiene,* Nov. 1989, 41(5): 512-520.

Kinosian. B.P., and J.M. Eisenber, "Cutting into cholesterol. Cost-effective alternatives for treating hypercholesterolemia," *Journal of the American Medical Association,* April 15, 1988, 259(15): 2249-54.

Kritchevsky, David, Charles Bonfield and James W. Anderson, eds., *Dietary Fiber.* (New York and London: Plenum Press, 1988).

Kritchevsky, David, and Charles Bonfield, *Dietary Fiber in Health and Disease.* (St. Paul, Minnesota: Eagan Press, 1995).

Kromhout, D., "Dietary fiber and 10-year mortality for coronary heart disease, cancer and all causes," *Lancet* 1982, 2: 518-22.

Leo, S. et al.,"Ulcerative colitis in remission: is it possible to predict the risk of relapse?" *Digestion,* 1989, 44(4): 217-21.

Lipsky, H., M. Gloger and W.H. Frishman, "Dietary Fiber for reducing blood cholesterol, *Journal of Clinical Pharmacology,* Aug. 1990, 30(8): 699-703.

Little. P., et al., "A controlled trial of low sodium, low fat, high fiber diet in treated hypersensitive patients" the efficacy of multiple dietary intervention," *Postgraduate Medical Journal* Aug. 1990, 66(778): 616-21.

Madar, Zacharia, and H. Selwyn Odes, *Dietary Fiber Research.* (Switzerland: Thur AG Offsetdruck, Pratteln, 1990).

Marckmann, P.; et al., "Low-Fat, High-Fiber Diet Favorably Affects Several Independent Risk Markers of Ischemic Heart Disease: Observations on Blood Lipids, Coagulation, and Fibrinolysis from a Trial of Middle-Aged Danes," *American Journal of Clinical Nutrition,* April, 1994, 59(4) 935-9.

Giovannucci E, et al., *Journal of the National Cancer Institute,* Jan, 1992, 15, 84(2):91-8

Michnovicz, Jon, M.D., Ph.D., *How to Reduce your Risk of Breast Cancer,* (New York: Warner Books, 1994).

Murray, Michael, N.D. and Joseph Pizzorno N.D., *Encyclopedia of Natural Medicine*. (Rocklin, California: Prima Publishing, 1991).

Neal, G.W., and T.K. Balm, "Synergistic effects of psyllium in the dietary treatment of hypercholesterolemia," *Southern Medical Journal,* Oct. 1990, 83(10): 1131-7.

McNamee, B., and V. Mansour-McNamee, *Dietary Fiber,* (Baltimore: Urban and Schwarzenberg, 1989).

Passwater, Richard A., Ph.D., *Cancer Prevention and Nutritional Therapies,* (New Canaan, Connecticut: Keats Publishing, 1993)..

Poynard et al., "Reduction of post-prandial insulin needs by pectin as assessed by the artificial pancreas in insulin-dependent diabetics," *Diabetes and Metabolism* 1982, 8(3): 187-9.

Fairweather-Tait S.J., and A.J. Wright, "The effect of sugar-beet fibre and wheat bran on iron and zinc absorption in rats," *British Journal of Nutrition,* Sept. 1990, 64(2): 547-52.

Trowell, Hugh, Denis Burkitt, and Kenneth Heaton, *Dietary Fibre, Fibre-Depleted Foods and Disease,* (London: Academic Press, 1985).

Prosky, Leon and Jonathan Devries, *Controlling Dietary Fiber in Food Products.* (New York: Van Nostrand Reinhold, 1992).

Rydning, A., et al., "Prophylactic effect of dietary fiber in duodenal ulcer disease," *Lancet,* 1982, 2:736.

Saldanha, L. G. *Pediatrics,* Nov. 1995, 96(5 Pt 2):994-7.

Scala, James, M.D., *Eating Right for a Bad Gut,* (New York: Penguin Books, 1990).

Schneider, T.F., and C. A. Edwards, eds., *Dietary Fibre, A Component of Food, Nutritional Function in Health and Disease,* (London: Springer-Verlag, 1992).

Smits, B.J., A.M. Whitehead and P. Prescott, "Lactulose in the treatment of symptomatic diverticular disease: a comparative study with high-fibre diet," *British Journal of Clinical Practice* Aug. 1990: 44(8): 314.

Snook, J., and H.A. Shepherd, "Bran supplementation in the treatment of irritable bowel syndrome," *Ailment-Pharmacology-Therapeutics* Oct. 1994, 8(5): 511-4.

Stephen, A.M., "Whole Grains—impact of consuming whole grains on physiological effects of dietary fiber and starch," Critical Review, *Food Science and Nutrition,* 1994, 34(5-6): 499-511.

Stoll, B.A., Oncology Department, St. Thomas' Hospital, London, UK., *Br J Cancer,* 1996, Mar;73(5):557-9.

Story, J.A., "Dietary Fiber and lipid metabolism," *Medical Aspects of Dietary Fiber,* (New York: Plenum Medical, 1980), 138.

U.S. Department of health and Human Services, *Healthy People 2000: National Health Promotion and Disease Prevention Objectives.* (Washington, D.C.: DHHS Publication, 1991), No. (PHS) 91-50213.

Williams C. L. et al., *Pediatrics,* Nov 1995, 96(5 Pt 2):985-8.